WALL-TO-WALL
THANKSGIVING

Kenneth Jernigan
Editor

Large Type Edition

A KERNEL BOOK
published by
NATIONAL FEDERATION OF THE BLIND

Table Of Contents

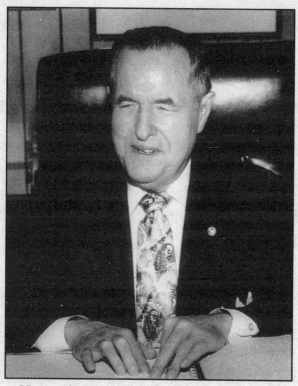

Kenneth Jernigan, President Emeritus
National Federation of the Blind

EDITOR'S INTRODUCTION

*M*ost American holidays have a double significance–what they are, and what they imply. New Year's Day, for instance, means just that, the beginning of another year. But it also means reviewing the past, planning for the future, and hoping to do better.

The Fourth of July commemorates the establishment of the nation. But over the years it has picked up a whole host of other meanings–everything from summer picnics and fireworks to how we should live and the current state of American values.

And then there is Thanksgiving, and also the present Kernel Book, the thirteenth in the series. When we started publishing the Kernel Books almost seven years ago, we didn't know how successful they would be, but our goal was to reach as many people as possible with true-life first-person stories told by blind persons themselves-how we raise children, hunt jobs, engage in courtship, get an education, go to church, cook a meal, meet friends, and do all of the other things that make up daily experience.

And we wanted to do it in such a way that the average member of the sighted public would read and be interested. The results have been better than we could possibly have hoped. More than three million of the Kernel Books are now in circulation, and I rarely travel anywhere in the country without being approached by someone who has read them and wants to talk about them or ask questions.

As to the present volume, *Wall-to-Wall Thanksgiving*, it is much like what has gone before. It tells about blind people as they live and work.

What does a blind boy do to earn summer spending money, and what do his sighted parents expect of him? What of the Viet Nam veteran who loses his sight in the war and comes home to build a new life? And what about the self-conscious child and young man with a little bit of sight who is ashamed of blindness and yet has to live with it?

What of the small details that come together to make the days that form the years–learning to ride a bicycle, cook a steak, read a book, get a job? This is what *Wall-to-Wall Thanksgiving* is about. I know the people who appear in its pages. They are friends of mine. Some have been my students. All of them are fellow participants in the work of the National Federation of the Blind.

If you wonder why so many of us give our time and effort to the Federation, it is because the Federation has played such an important part in making life better for us. In fact, the National Federation of the Blind has done more than any other single thing to improve the quality of life for blind persons in the twentieth century. It is blind persons coming together to help each other and do for themselves.

That does not mean that we don't want or need help from our sighted friends and associates, for we do. But it does mean that we think we ought to try to help ourselves before we ask others for assistance. And we should also give as well as take. All of this is what the National Federation of the Blind stands for and means.

I have edited the Kernel Books from the beginning, and I have contributed a story to each of them. My present offering deals with help I have received from sighted people. Sometimes my reactions have been appropriate and mature; sometimes not. As you read what I have written, you will see that my views have changed as I have grown older. Perhaps the title of my submission, *Don't Throw the Nickel*, sums it up.

As to the title of this thirteenth volume in the Kernel Book series, *Wall-to-Wall Thanksgiving*, it is taken from the story of the same name by Barbara Pierce. But like the holidays, it has more than a single meaning. With all of the difficulties we have had and with all of the problems we currently experience, we who are blind have more reason for Thanksgiving now than ever before in history.

Unlike many in today's society, we do not think of ourselves as victims, and we feel that our future is bright with promise. That is so because we intend to work to make it so, and because more and more sighted people are joining our cause and helping make it happen.

I hope you will enjoy this book and that it will give you worthwhile information.

Kenneth Jernigan
Baltimore, Maryland
1997

Why Large Type

The type size in this book is 14 point for two important reasons: One, because typesetting of 14 point or larger complies with federal standards for the printing of materials for visually impaired readers, and we want to show you exactly what type size is necessary for people with limited sight.

The second reason is that many of our friends and supporters have asked us to print our paperback books in 14 point type so they too can easily read them. Many people with limited sight do not use Braille. We hope that by printing this book in a larger type than customary, many more people will be able to benefit from it.

Don't Throw The Nickel

by Kenneth Jernigan

When is it appropriate for a blind person to accept help from a sighted person, and when is it not? If the offer is rejected, how can it be done without causing embarrassment or hurt feelings? Since most sighted people are well-disposed toward the blind, these are very real questions–questions that I as a blind person have faced all of my life. As you might imagine, my answers to them have changed as I have grown older and gained experience.

When I was a teen-ager, filled with the typical self-consciousness of adolescence, I frequently rode city buses. This was in Nashville, Tennessee. The school for the blind, where I was a student, was located on the southern edge of the city, and I liked to go downtown. Incidentally, in those days a bus ride cost a nickel, as did a lot of other things–a hamburger, a Coca-Cola, an order of French fries, a full-size candy bar, a double-dip of ice cream, and much else.

But back to the matter at hand. One day I was standing on the corner waiting for a bus when an elderly woman approached me and said, "Here, son, I'll help you." She then put a nickel into my hand.

I could tell that she was elderly because of her voice. There was quite a crowd at the bus stop, and I felt acute embarrassment. I tried to give the nickel back to her, but she moved out of my way and kept saying, "No, that's all right."

Everybody at the bus stop ceased talking, and my frustration mounted. Each time I stepped toward her to try to give back the nickel, she moved out of my way. It must have been quite a spectacle, me with my hand extended holding the nickel, and the woman weaving and dodging to avoid me. Finally, in absolute exasperation, I threw the nickel as far as I could down the street.

That was over fifty years ago, but the memory is still clear. Once the woman had placed the nickel in my hand, there was really no way I could have given it back. If I had simply and quietly accepted it and thanked her, very little notice would have been taken.

As it was, I created quite a show. The elderly woman, who was only trying to help me, was undoubtedly embarrassed, and I did little to improve the image of blindness. Instead, I did the exact opposite. Any notions the group at the bus stop had about the helplessness and immaturity of the blind were magnified and reinforced.

Ten years later, when I was in my twenties, I was teaching at the California training center for the blind in the San Francisco Bay area. One of my principal duties was to help newly blind persons learn how to deal maturely with loss of sight and the attitudes of the public about blindness.

Late one afternoon, after a particularly hard day, I was leaving the center to go home. When I came to the corner to cross the street, an elderly man (he sounded as if he might be in his eighties) approached me and said, "I'll help you across the street."

"No, thanks," I said. "I can make it just fine." I was polite but firm.

"I'll help," he repeated, and took my arm. As I have already said, it had been a hard day.

I made no discourteous response, but I speeded up my pace as we crossed the street.

Clearly the man could not keep up, and if I am to be honest, I knew that he couldn't. He released my arm and said with a hurt tone, "I was only trying to help."

When I got to the other side of the street, I came to a complete stop and said to myself, "Are you really so insecure about your blindness after a hard day you can't afford to be kind to somebody who was only trying to help you?"

As with the nickel-throwing incident, there was a lesson to be learned. I should have accepted the man's offer of help, and should have done it graciously. We would both have profited, each feeling that he had done the other a kindness. As it was, both of us experienced pain, even if only a little and even if only temporarily.

By the time another ten years had passed, I was in my thirties and directing programs for the blind in the state of Iowa. My job required me to do a great deal of traveling, and one day when I was checking into a hotel, a bellman carried my bag to my room. As he was leaving, I gave him a tip.

"Oh, no," he said, "I couldn't take a tip from you. I'm a Christian."

Unlike what I did in the other situations I have described, I did not refuse or resist. I simply thanked him and let it go at that. Of course, I might have tried to get him to change his mind, but I didn't think it would be productive. And besides, I didn't feel so insecure or unsure of myself that I needed to prove either to him or me that I was equal.

On another occasion in Iowa, I was giving a talk to a Sunday School class, and when the time came for questions, a woman said: "How do you help one of them?" I assumed that she was asking me what the proper way was for a sighted person to help a blind person, but just to make sure I asked her to explain.

She said: "The other day I tried to help a blind man across the street, and he shook my hand off of his arm and told me to go to hell." I asked her what she would have done if a sighted person had been rude to her.

I said something to this effect: "You shouldn't hesitate to offer help to a blind person in crossing a street or in any other way you think appropriate. After all, the blind person may need your help. How are you to know if you don't ask?

Whether the help is needed or not, most blind persons (just as would be the case with most sighted persons) will appreciate the offer and treat you courteously. A few will be ill-tempered or rude. I would suggest that you treat such people exactly the way you would a sighted person who is rude to you. The main thing is not to feel awkward about it. If you wonder whether a blind person needs help, ask. Then, if the person says no, let it go at that.

So far, I have talked about help that has been courteously offered and probably should have been accepted. But what about the other kind? Blind people don't have a monopoly on rudeness or bad manners. Sighted people are human, too.

I think of a time when I was standing on a street corner in Des Moines, minding my own business and waiting for a friend. A big husky fellow with the momentum of a freight train came along and scooped me up without ever even pausing. "Come on, buddy," he said, as he grabbed my arm, "I'll help you across the street."

As it so happened, I didn't want to cross that street. I was going in another direction. But he didn't ask. And he wouldn't listen when I tried to tell him. He just kept walking and dragging me with him.

In the circumstances, I planted my feet and resisted–and I should have. All of us, whether blind or sighted, owe courtesy and consideration to each other, and in this case I was being treated like a none-too-intelligent child. No, worse than that–for children are rarely manhandled in public.

Not long ago I entered an elevator, and a man standing next to me reached out and placed his hand on my arm, between me and the elevator door, in a protective manner. He probably felt that I might lean into the door as it was closing or that I might have difficulty when the door opened. It was a protective gesture, totally inappropriate but meant to be helpful. He would have been shocked at the thought of behaving that way toward a sighted adult passenger, but in my case he saw no impropriety.

When the door opened, the man restrained me with his hand and said, "Wait. You can't go yet." Since I was standing immediately next to the door and since there was no traffic outside, it is hard to know why he felt I should wait. Maybe he thought I should take a moment to get my bearings, or maybe it was simply more of the protectiveness. Who knows?

He treated me very much as he would have treated a small child. How should I have reacted? It all depends on how insistent and how obtrusive he was. There is something to be said for restraint and not hurting other people's feelings, but there is also something to be said for recognizing when enough is enough.

In what I am about to say next, I am not just talking about persons who are totally blind but also about those who now see so poorly that they cannot function the way a sighted person does—persons who may be losing sight and who may be having trouble accepting it. I am also speaking to relatives.

As I have already indicated, most blind people appreciate help when it is offered.

When a blind person is walking through a crowd or down the street with someone else and trying to carry on a conversation, it is easier to take the other person's arm. This is true even if the blind person is quite capable of traveling alone.

All of us like to do things for ourselves, but there are times when refusing to take an arm that is offered constitutes the very opposite of independence for a blind person. If, for instance, a blind person is walking with a sighted person through a crowded restaurant, the sensible thing to do is to take the sighted person's arm and go to the table without fuss or bother.

As will be seen, my views about independence and help from others have changed over the years. Probably the single most important factor in helping me come to my present notions has been the National Federation of the Blind. Having chapters in every state and almost every community of any size, the Federation is the nation's oldest and largest organization of blind persons.

As it is with me, so it is with thousands of other blind people throughout the country.

We work together to help each other and ourselves. We give assistance to parents of blind children, to blind college students, to the newly blind, and to blind persons who are trying to find employment. Above all, the Federation teaches a new way of thought about blindness.

We want to take the mystery out of blindness. Mostly, we who are blind are very much like you. We work and play, hope and dream, laugh and cry–just like you. We need opportunity, not pity. And we are willing to do for ourselves. That doesn't mean that we don't want or need help from our sighted friends and relatives, for we do. All of us (whether blind or not) depend on each other and need mutual help and assistance.

This is the message of the National Federation of the Blind, and it has made a great difference in my life. If I had to sum up my personal philosophy in a single sentence, it would probably be this: Do all you can to help yourself before you call on others; try to make life better for those around you; and don't throw nickels.

Boy, Was I Bamboozled

by Bruce Gardner

*T*oday Bruce Gardner is a successful practicing attorney. He is also President of the National Federation of the Blind of Arizona. From early childhood Bruce and two older brothers had very limited eyesight. Even so, they did not think of themselves as blind and often went to great lengths to pretend they could see. In his story, "Boy, Was I Bamboozled," Bruce tells us what it was like for an eight-year-old boy to learn that he was going blind. Here is what he has to say:

I remember when I first learned that I was going blind. I was about eight years old when my friend said, "Look at the jackrabbit under the mesquite tree." I said, "What mesquite tree?" Not only could I not see the rabbit, I could not see the tree.

My mother called us all in and set us in a row on the couch to play a game. She held up flash cards, and one at a time we tried to see how far away she could stand and have us still read the cards. I could not read the flash cards without holding them up to my face.

When she took me to the eye doctor to be examined he said, "Well, it's another one." I was the third in our family of nine children to be diagnosed as having macular degeneration. I had no central vision and could therefore see no details, but only light and dark, general shapes and movement.

I grew up being embarrassed and ashamed of my blindness. We avoided the word *blind* because of its negative connotations. *Visually impaired* was much better. After all, lots of people wore glasses and had imperfect vision, and that was okay. But if you crossed that invisible line into the realm of blindness, then all the myths were heaped upon you. Therefore, growing up I was not blind–I just couldn't see. Boy, was I bamboozled!

My parents had already spent years and large sums of the family's scarce resources taking my two older brothers to countless specialists searching for a cure. By the time I was diagnosed, hope for a cure was wearing thin. Therefore, I was not taken to as many eye specialists as were my older brothers.

But, I do vividly remember as a little boy going to one eye specialist and hearing the doctor tell my parents that there was nothing he could do for my eyes. The doctor said that because my blindness was undoubtedly hereditary, they should make sure that I never got married or had children.

I remember my mother sobbing and her feeling that somehow it was her fault that I was blind. The clear message from the doctor was that it would have been better if I had not been born. And of course, I absorbed that message. Boy, was I bamboozled!

As a boy I watched the show "Mr. Magoo." I outwardly laughed at the bumbling blind man, but inside I hurt. Blind people were fumbling, bumbling Mr. Magoos or helpless dependents, who sold pencils on the street corner. Half of me refused to admit that I was blind, because blindness meant helplessness.

The other half of me would reply, "Oh, you think you are not blind! Well then, look across the room and identify who just walked in. And pick up that book and read it if you're not blind. Don't kid yourself. You're blind. You are nothing more than a fumbling, bumbling Mr. Magoo."

Of course I did not want anyone to know of my blindness, so I would do crazy things to appear "normal." It was like playing "blind man's bluff." I would pretend to be reading a magazine in the barber shop or a doctor's office and turn the pages after the appropriate passage of time, or loiter in lobbies outside what I hoped were the rest rooms (sometimes in increasing discomfort) in order to identify a man, and then observe which door he went through so I could follow him into the correct rest room.

It was unthinkable for me to ask for directions for fear the rest room was close by when I asked, because then they would know that I could not see. I would rather be thought of as unfriendly or stuck-up and rude than let people know I did not see or recognize them. Boy, was I bamboozled!

I was in third grade when I learned I was going blind. From third grade until seventh grade I did not do any reading. My mother read to me at home, and my teachers did not call on me to read at school. I did not see how words were spelled but only heard how they were pronounced. Since words are often not spelled the way they are pronounced, my spelling is–shall we say–creative.

In seventh grade I got a magnifying glass that was strong enough for me to read a little. The focal point was about the length of my nose, so when I read I could only see about a word at a time. That is, if it was a short word. If it was a longer word, I could not see both ends at the same time.

I would get my nose black when I read back something I had written because I had to be so close to the paper. Of course, reading in this manner was extremely slow and tiring. Needless to say, I should have been taught Braille, but I was not given that opportunity.

After all, I still had a little vision and could *read* print. Never mind that with Braille I could have read ten times faster and for extended periods of time. To read Braille would have meant admitting that I was blind, and that was unthinkable. Boy, was I bamboozled!

In high school I signed up for advanced placement English. I was in all respects qualified for the advanced course. However, the teacher told me that I could not take the class because I was blind. She said that there was simply too much reading and that I would not be able to keep up.

She told me that I should take the bare minimum of English classes. She knew nothing about talking books or Braille. She was well-intentioned, but uninformed. She was also convincing. So, I followed her advice and took the minimum of English classes in both high school and college. In fact, I even took a philosophy class in college because it gave English credit without being an *English* class. Boy, was I bamboozled!

It was not until I was in law school that I realized how unwise I had been. More English courses would have helped me a great deal– both in law school and in the practice of law.

Thankfully, when I was 21 the National Federation of the Blind found me and helped me learn the truth about blindness. I now know that with opportunity and training, blindness need not be a tragedy. I now know that it is respectable to be blind.

I will forever be grateful to the National Federation of the Blind for sharing with me the truth about my blindness and helping to heal the hurt and remove the shame of a little blind boy who had been bamboozled.

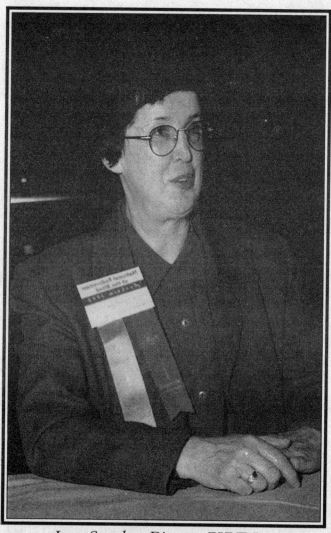

Joyce Scanlan, Director, BLIND Inc.

Lessons From The Charcoal Pit

by Joyce Scanlan

Today Joyce Scanlan is the director of one of the National Federation of the Blind's regional training centers for blind adults. On a daily basis she helps her blind students come to believe that they can live productive lives. From personal experience she knows that this belief is hard to come by. She knows that it has to be painstakingly built, often in small and unexpected ways, and that we as blind people must encourage each other.

In "Lessons From the Charcoal Pit," Joyce tells of a pivotal event in her own journey to belief. Although I happened to be one giving the encouragement in the situation she describes, it could just as well have been any of a hundred others, because this is what we do in the National Federation of the Blind. Here is Joyce's story:

Growing up in the state of North Dakota I knew what isolation and loneliness were. I knew what being on my own meant. I knew how to fight my battles (or I thought I did), for I was an independent thinker and considered myself highly informed on all matters. I had received a college education past the master's degree level and had been successfully employed as a teacher.

I was not blind; I only had a visual problem. In my opinion no one knew I was anything but sighted, so what a rude awakening I had when I suddenly learned that I was destined to lose my remaining sight and would probably become totally blind. Suddenly my bubble burst.

My goal had always been to become a college English professor, but when I faced blindness, that goal became something seemingly unachievable. My livelihood, career plans, and independence all appeared to vanish.

It was not a happy time. In 1970 I had hit bottom. Then, the National Federation of the Blind Convention came to Minneapolis, where I was then living, and I went. I went because a friend practically dragged me there after I had run out of excuses. That was almost three decades ago.

The convention was indeed a life-changing experience. Spending four or five days meeting blind teachers from all over the country, and discussing interesting topics about blindness with all kinds of well-informed people proved to me that I had been doing everything wrong and needed to make some drastic changes in my life. My style of going it alone had not worked and would never work. The Federation had a lot to teach me.

I remember vividly to this day an evening I spent with Kenneth Jernigan twenty-four years ago. It was, perhaps, a little thing–but, it changed my life. At the time, Dr. Jernigan was President of the National Federation of the Blind, and I was attending a training seminar over Labor Day weekend.

The first evening, when we were all going out to dinner together, someone suggested we go to a place called the Charcoal Pit. We were told that we would be able to select and grill our own steaks. I said I didn't like the idea because I had never before grilled a steak to my liking. Dr. Jernigan very calmly said, "Oh well, I'll help you." I was suddenly terrified, for both of us were totally blind, and I didn't see how we could do it.

I prayed that, when we got to the Charcoal Pit, he would have forgotten what I had said. Of course, that didn't happen. He immediately escorted me to the refrigerators, where all the steaks were kept. He was so enthusiastic and seemed to be having such fun that I began to enjoy the venture myself.

With the steak selected, a plate, and a long fork in hand, we approached the big pit. He said, "Now throw your steak out there; just toss it out there." I did, thinking all the time about losing the steak forever in the fire.

After a short while, Dr. Jernigan said, "All right, reach out with your fork and find the steak and put it on the plate." I did. Then he showed me how to turn the steak over. I was so relieved that he had done it, so I wouldn't have to touch that hot meat.

However, he flipped the steak back and said to me, "Now you do it." I should have known he wouldn't let me off so easy. Then we grilled the steak on the other side, and I became more comfortable handling it.

I ate the steak and enjoyed it, too. Everyone was having such a good time, and for the first time I actually enjoyed a steak that I had cooked. Then Dr. Jernigan asked me to grill a second steak for him. It must have been okay because he ate it and didn't complain. I learned much about myself, about leadership, and about dealing with blindness just from that one experience.

I'm glad there is a National Federation of the Blind. I know that, when I was a child, when I was in college, when I was teaching, and when I was struggling to deal with blindness, other blind people were busy founding a movement to help me and others like me. I'm grateful and pleased that they did that. But even more, I feel a strong sense of responsibility to do as they did to keep this movement strong and vibrant for the next generation of blind people, who will have much less struggle than I did because of the work that we have done.

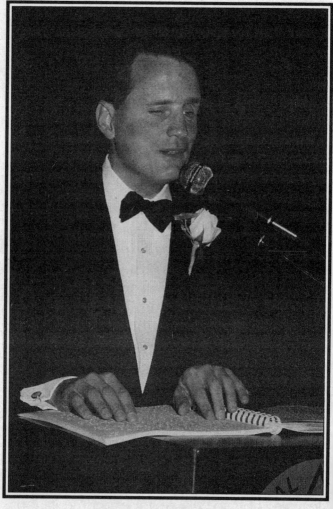

Marc Maurer, President
National Federation of the Blind

Concerning Books, Lawn Mowers, And Bus Rides

by Marc Maurer

Marc Maurer is President of the National Federation of the Blind. As regular Kernal Book readers know, he has been blind since birth. In this story he reflects upon his own experience growing up as a blind child–from how he felt at age six when he came home from the hospital totally blind after surgery intended to restore his eyesight not only failed but also caused him to lose the tiny amount of vision he had to his determined effort to be a fully contributing member of the family. Here is what he has to say:

When I was growing up, it seemed to me that my parents were always telling me what to do. Now that I am an adult with children of my own, I am very frequently required to remind my children to do the things they know they must. Sometimes they pay attention, but sometimes they don't.

The growing up years are the time for learning how to behave, for experimentation, and for seeking maturity. During this period parents are faced with many decisions—decisions that won't wait: What discipline should be imposed? How much freedom can the children manage? What experiences should they have? How much direction can effectively be given? And what is the proper balance between encouraging independence and maintaining sufficient control to guard against disaster? Too much protection can stifle initiative, and too little can lead to ruin. This basic set of considerations is as important for sighted parents raising blind children as it is for those raising sighted children.

I was born blind. However, I had a tiny amount of residual vision. Nobody ever told me that I was blind, so I didn't realize it until I was five.

My parents loved me, and they wanted very much for me to be a normal, healthy child. When I was six, they took me to an eye doctor for a new kind of operation, but it didn't work. Worse than that. As a result of it, I became totally blind.

For several weeks I was moody and despondent. Late one hot summer night I was sitting on my father's lap on the front porch swing. He struck a match. The sudden flare startled me, and I jumped. I had been able to see the light of the flame. All of us wondered what it meant, and my father hoped fervently that I would be able to regain the use of my eyes. But this was not to be. I would remain blind, and we must decide how to manage. None of us knew what to do, but my parents were determined that my blindness should limit me as little as possible.

During the next summer (between my first and second grade school years), my mother taught me to read Braille. Reading was part of the accepted pattern in our family, and my mother expected me to read as much as she expected every other child in our family to read. But there wasn't much Braille material available. During the winter, while I was attending the school for the blind, Braille books were fairly easy to come by. But during the summer, the three months that I spent at home with my family, Braille was scarce.

One year somebody put my name on a list to receive the Braille edition of *My Weekly Reader*. It came in a big, brown envelope about a foot across and fifteen inches high. The magazine was about twenty-five pages long, and I looked forward to getting it.

In 1960, Dr. Kenneth Jernigan established a library for the blind in Iowa, my home state. My father read about the library in the paper, and he asked me if I would like to sign up to borrow Braille books. I told him that I most certainly would. The next time my father drove through Des Moines, he stopped at the library to enroll me as a borrower. Soon afterward, the first of the books arrived in the mail.

The packages I received contained three or four volumes. Braille books can be long. *Gone With the Wind* is ten volumes, but Charles Dickens's *A Christmas Carol* is only one. Each volume I got from the library was about twelve inches square, and about three inches thick. They came to me wrapped in heavy brown paper tied with string.

I very carefully untied the string and folded the paper–both must be saved for reuse in shipping the books back to the library. Books for the blind travel through the mail postage free. Inside the front cover of each volume was a mailing label containing the address of the library. The label was to be pasted on the package to return it to the library. Storing the books, caring for them, and seeing that they were packaged to be mailed back were my responsibility.

When the books were ready for shipment, sometimes my mother would take them to the post office for me in the car. However, this was not always convenient. Sometimes I would load the bundles onto my red wagon and haul them to the post office. The people in the post office never seemed very glad to see me. They appeared to me to be stern and official. I was glad to get out of there, but I wanted more books, so I was willing to face the officialdom of the postal service.

Because the books arrived by mail, planning was required to insure that there was always a supply on hand. I could get two (or sometimes three) books at a time. If I read them all and sent them back, I would have no books until the new shipment arrived. Consequently, I worked out a revolving book loan system with the library.

In the summers in the middle of Iowa, there were certain activities for entertainment. I could sometimes go swimming, but the pool was more than a mile and a half walk from my house. Occasionally there were picnics, but not often. There were television and radio, and sometimes there were rambles in the park or the woods.

However, in those days I did not believe a blind person could travel through the park or the woods alone. My excursions on the nature trails were restricted to times when a friend or a brother could go with me. My parents bought me a bicycle built for two, which I could ride if I found somebody to take the front seat.

Then, there were the projects to make a little money. We collected empty soda bottles because you could get two cents a piece for them if they weren't chipped. One summer my brothers and I started a lawn mowing business. The local newspaper agreed to help kids try to find summer employment by publishing ads for them at no charge. We accepted.

My father told me that I could use the lawn mower as long as I maintained it in good repair, bought the gas and oil for it, and kept our own yard mowed. We got about half a dozen regular customers, who wanted their lawns mowed every two weeks.

When they called, we would gas up the lawn mower and take it to cut the grass. We liked to do it in the mornings–because it was cooler. But we would work any time. We wanted the cash that the mowing produced.

My brother was small enough that he couldn't push the mower very well, but he could guide it. I pushed, and he steered. When the mowing had been completed, we both raked the grass clippings and bagged them for the trash collector. We charged four dollars for small lawns and five for large ones.

It may not sound like much to those who have become accustomed to today's inflated allowances and pay for teen-agers, but we could earn twenty dollars in a day if we were lucky. And that seemed like a lot. To me it still does.

All of us in the Maurer family did housework. After the inside chores, each of us was assigned yard work for an hour. Once we were directed to tuck-point the foundation of our home. When the mortar between the bricks gets old and loose, it must be scraped out and replaced with new concrete. Of course, not all of the mortar deteriorates. If it did, the foundation would collapse.

The tuck-pointing process repairs surface damage. It is a tedious and messy job. Each morning for several weeks, we mixed a batch of mortar and applied it to the foundation, replacing damaged concrete in the joints between all of the exposed bricks.

Even with all of the activities I have described, I had a lot of free time in the summers. I filled it reading. The library was my friend, but it was a mysterious friend—one that I had never met. I wanted to know more about it.

I asked my mother if I could visit the library in Des Moines, forty miles from our home in Boone; and she agreed. Two of my brothers and I decided that we would take the Greyhound Bus to get there, and I began saving pennies for the trip. The bus ticket cost $3.30 for adults and $1.65 for children. I qualified for the adult fare, but my younger brothers could get the cheaper rate.

It took me quite a while to get the money together. This particular trip was planned before I had come upon the lawn mowing business. My father might give me fifty cents a week for my allowance, and there might be some other money from the collection of the soda bottles, but that was about it.

After saving for weeks, we had the money; and we headed for the local bus station-a counter at Eddie's newspaper shop. But when we got there, Eddie told us there had been a fare increase. The spare change we had saved for emergencies had to go. We spent all our money on bus tickets.

The bus ride from Boone to Des Moines took about an hour. When we arrived at the Des Moines bus station, we discovered that it was only a short walk to the library for the blind. I was delighted with all of the books, and with the friendliness of the staff members there. They said I could browse to my heart's content and pick out anything I wanted.

After a while, I found a good book, and I started to read. One of the staff members brought me a chair and asked if I needed anything else. I said that I did not, and I just kept reading.

After a time my brothers got bored with the library. They are sighted, and they cannot read Braille. I was the oldest (thirteen or fourteen at the time), so I was in charge. My brothers asked me if they could visit the state capitol building, and I told them they could. They disappeared and were gone for hours. I didn't care at all; I had the books. Perhaps it is just as well that my mother didn't know about the nature of my supervision that day.

Late in the afternoon, my brothers returned; and we headed back to the bus station. All of us were quite hungry. We had neglected to bring lunch, and we didn't have any money to buy any. We had spent all we had on the bus tickets. But the ride home was cheerful, and I carried a book with me to read on the bus.

It was the first trip away from home that I ever planned. I wished that I had thought about the lunch. But despite this mistake, I was satisfied. I had seen the library, and I had a book. Not only that. I had the prospect of hundreds and thousands more.

My parents required me to work, gave me independence, and taught me to read. They let me know in a thousand ways that I was a cherished member of the family. They insisted that I make contributions, and they made it perfectly clear that the standard of behavior and the quality of work required would be no less for me than for the other children in the family. As I look back from the perspective of manhood and with children of my own, this is the way it should have been.

In the National Federation of the Blind we are committed to help blind children get the best education their minds can take. Building the right future demands education, a spirit of self-reliance, and the balance to know when to guide and when to keep hands off.

For those of us who have reached adulthood, the pattern of life is established. However, for the children the dreams for the future can be as broad as our imagination and our commitment permit. We believe in our children, and whenever we can find a way to do it, we will put a book into their hands.

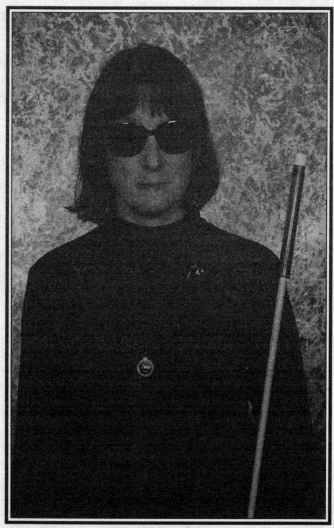

Barbara Walker

CHILDREN, FRUITCAKE, AND RECTANGLES

by Barbara Walker

Barbara Walker is no stranger to readers of previous Kernel Books–her sensitive and thought-provoking stories having appeared in a number of them. Here she reflects on the key ingredients of her own childhood, which enabled her to find her place in the world–as a leader in her community, her church, and the National Federation of the Blind. Here is what she has to say:

When my son John, at the age of three, said he wanted some fruitcake that had been in the refrigerator for quite awhile, I said: "Just a minute, please. I need to see what kind of shape it's in." His response was immediate: "It's in a rectangle shape, and I want some." Somehow, his response got me to thinking about my own childhood.

I have always been blind. My sister, Laurie, is also blind. Our older brother, Lani, isn't. There was, to our parents' knowledge, no history of blindness in our family.

Discussing my sister's case, the doctors said they didn't know the cause of blindness, but thought there was probably a one in a thousand chance of recurrence. Since I arrived–blind–fourteen months later, either I'm one in a thousand, or they didn't know what they were talking about. All of us are now grown, married, and have children–none of whom is blind.

Our parents knew nothing about blindness. They struggled with stereotypes as all of us do, but their hope for us was the same as that for our brother–that we would eventually be contributing and fulfilled adults, no longer needing or wanting to live under their care.

My sister, from what I remember my mother's telling me, crawled, walked, and talked at about the same time as neighbor kids her age. She ran away from home more than once while still in diapers, handled everything she could get to, was adept with her fingers, questioned incessantly, and insisted on a prominent place in her world.

I, on the other hand, neither walked nor talked until I was about two, showed little visible evidence that I was particularly curious about my environment, and was clumsy and awkward with my hands and body–breaking many things with which I came into contact.

As toddlers and preschoolers, we continued to show contrasts. Laurie, at age two, walked along the piano reaching up to pick out melodies on the keyboard. She generally chose gentle play–interacting with others, real or imaginary–and was afraid of high slides, going on carnival rides, and the like.

I loved rough play–wrestling, running hard, swinging and/or climbing high, flipping over and off of bars, throwing and catching balls, etc.–and I loved high slides, carnival rids, and the like.

Mom, the more verbally expressive of our parents, said there were many times when she didn't understand how we would or could do things, and it scared her to have us try. But she didn't stand in our way. She learned Braille so that we could correspond privately.

She persistently went to bat for us when we were left out or mistreated–not in ways that made us dependent upon her, but in ways that preserved respect and dignity for everyone, and provided us with experience in everything from fielding questions to finding alternative methods for doing things ordinarily done with the use of sight.

Dad showed his acceptance of us in other ways. He showed us how things worked. He pointed out nonvisual qualities of things generally perceived visually, like the contrasting cool and hot pavement where his shadow passed. He made us doll cribs and a playhouse. Dad also took me fishing and encouraged my interests in competitive sports.

My sister and I were given hands-on experiences whenever their availability and our interests coincided. I was a very shy child, and sometimes my self-consciousness prevented me from taking full advantage of these opportunities. If Laurie was along, I generally asked her later about whatever we had seen, and she would explain it in detail–sometimes creating a replica to show me.

Underlying all of these things were our parents' respect for us as people and their encouragement toward our finding a place in society–not a pigeonhole created by them or anyone else, but a place we could earn as others do. That genuine attitude of respect and affirmation of our worth and dignity did more than all the experiences and skills combined in allowing us to grow and become contributing members of society.

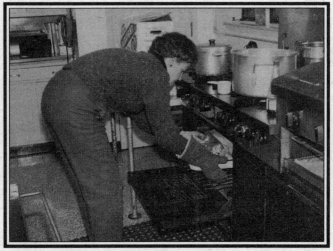

Barbara Pierce

THE WALL-TO-WALL THANKSGIVING

by Barbara Pierce

Barbara Pierce is no stranger to Kernel Book readers, having appeared in these pages frequently. The remarkable thing about her current story is that it records truly unremarkable events–the sort that occur regularly in any typical household. Read her heartwarming account of her young family's efforts to celebrate traditional American holidays while living in London and see if you don't come to believe that we who are blind are people–just like you in more ways than not. Here is what she has to say:

Almost twenty years ago my English-professor husband Bob; our three children (Steven, nine; Anne, six; and Margaret, just four); and I packed up and moved to London for the school year. Bob was to teach our college's London semester program during the fall semester. (This would give our American students the experience of studying and living in England.) Bob would then spend the spring doing his own scholarship during his sabbatical leave. The children, including little Margy, would all attend school, and I planned to keep house, try my hand at writing a book, and spend time getting to know the members of the National Federation of the Blind of the United Kingdom.

We were lucky to find a small house to rent in one of the outlying suburbs. The elementary school was nearby, as were the shops where I would spend a good deal of time and the tube station from which Bob would leave for central London every morning. Best of all, our next-door neighbor had a niece around the corner who was willing to baby-sit for us during the evenings when Bob and I went to the theater with his students.

We settled in easily, and the shopkeepers became accustomed to my long white cane, American accent, two-wheeled shopping trolley, and occasional gaggle of children. Expeditions to the butcher, greengrocer, chemist, and grocery shop were easier and faster without the youngsters, but so were cleaning the house and writing. Besides, the girls especially loved to "go to the shops" with me, so we quickly became an institution in the neighborhood.

By late October the whole family had become acclimatized to life in London. The children had made friends and were developing English accents. I was resigned to washing school uniforms in the bath tub on the days when I didn't go to the laundromat. And Bob had established a warm relationship with his students.

We decided that on the Saturday before Halloween we should invite the whole class to supper. They had tickets to a Saturday matinee performance of a Shakespeare play, so it would be easy for all of them to come back to the house together at the close of the performance.

I didn't even consider attending the play that day. After all, somebody had to prepare supper for that crowd, and I didn't think that the baby-sitter and the children would get very far picking up the living room, much less setting out the food I had prepared.

Steven had been somewhat disappointed at missing Halloween at home in Ohio with its costumes and trick or treating, so we decided to do what we could to celebrate this important annual rite of American childhood with our party. I made a big chocolate cake and let the children tint the butter frosting a shocking shade of orange. We managed to find candy corn and witches with which to decorate our masterpiece.

But the real triumph of the meal was to be the loaf of homemade bread. I had decided that, considering the small rooms of our house, I would have to settle for feeding the students sandwiches and potato chips– "crisps" in London.

I arranged a large tray of sliced meats and cheeses and another of fresh vegetables and dip. I bought several sorts of rolls and small interesting loaves. But in the center of the table was a large loaf of potato bread in the shape of a jack-o-lantern, complete with eyes, eye brows, ears, nose, and mouth full of snaggly teeth.

Anne was regretful that I would not agree to make the bread orange or allow her to frost the finished loaf with the left-over icing from the cake. But despite its shortcomings in the eyes of the children, our pumpkin was the hit of the evening.

Bob and the students were late getting home from the play, and in the interim a glass of liquid got spilled by one of the children, but it hardly dampened the upholstery or the spirits of the party.

The students were delighted to be in a home with children to play with. And you would have thought I had prepared a banquet for them instead of a simple supper.

When I saw them at the theater during the early weeks of November, they continued to talk wistfully about the fun they had had with our family.

As Thanksgiving approached, I began to realize that I was going to have to do something about the holiday. It isn't celebrated in England, of course, and our American students were beginning to feel homesick at the prospect of being so far away from family for the holiday. But having sixteen students in for sandwiches and finger food on paper plates and doing a complete Thanksgiving dinner for them were two very different things.

For one, we had six plates and about as many sets of silverware. There was almost no counter space in the kitchen, and though the stove had four burners, the oven was half the size of my oven at home. But it was clear that, problems or no, Thanksgiving was going to be celebrated in memorable style in the Pierce home that year. I asked each student to bring a plate and silverware for each person that he or she was bringing to dinner, and I invited them all to bring along some contribution of food.

Meanwhile I had managed to find one of those large foil disposable roasting pans in a local department store. Much to my relief, when I got it home, it actually fit into my oven. I took it off to the butcher and asked him to get me the largest turkey that would fit into the pan.

He did so, and he even agreed to keep it in his freezer for me until I was ready to cope with it. The day before the Feast, as the children began calling that Thanksgiving, I stopped to make sure that the butcher had moved the turkey from the freezer into his cooler for me. He assured me that he had and that it would be thawed for me in the morning. Relieved of that nagging worry, I went home to get on with my preparations.

When I went into the kitchen to begin dinner, I discovered to my horror that the oven would not light. Here was a nightmare indeed. Luckily the Gas Board was not about to shut down for a long holiday weekend, so they promised that someone would be around first thing in the morning to see about the cooker.

My dreams were filled that night with catastrophes in which I was trying to roast turkeys over matches. But in the morning we experienced a whole series of miracles. First, the Gas Board man turned up early. Second, he discovered that there was nothing seriously wrong with the stove, and he could and did fix it immediately. The third event took a little longer to resolve itself into a miracle. It began by looking remarkably like a catastrophe.

While I stayed home to deal with the stove and the other preparations, Bob took the children with him to do the last minute shopping, including picking up the turkey. I was busy finishing the stuffing when I realized that in the distance I was hearing Margy crying as the Pierce parade drew near our house.

I raced to the door to see what the trouble was. I could hardly believe the news; the butcher had not in fact transferred the turkey to the cooler as he had alleged; when Bob handed it to me, it was eighteen pounds of rock-hard meat–giblets and neck firmly tucked inside the body cavity. Though Margy was the only one actually in tears, all three children were certain that Thanksgiving had just crash landed in the butcher's freezer.

There are moments when a parent has no choice but to set aside anger, frustration, and anxiety and simply rally all available reserves in the emergency. I dried Margy's tears and assured everybody that the day could be saved.

Then the turkey and I retired to the kitchen sink for some close communion with warm water. It was not the correct way to defrost poultry, but I told myself that, if I could just pry the giblets out and pack the stuffing in quickly, I could get the bird on to roast before anything nasty began growing in the meat.

It worked. By late afternoon we were ready for the Feast, and the students began to arrive, bearing an unusual collection of dishes. Including several strays picked up by various people along the way, twenty-three happy Americans eventually sat down to Thanksgiving dinner. In fact, we sat down all over the house. The living and dining room floors were covered with bodies, and six of us sat on the steps to the second story. We had a marvelous time! The food was delicious, and the fellowship was unforgettable. I don't even remember the clean-up.

Everyone had so much fun that we decided to do it again the following year when we were all back in the United States. By then many of the students had graduated, but they returned to Oberlin for Thanksgiving and a reunion of the London semester group. In some ways the two celebrations were very different. .

There were no crises the second time around. I managed to come up with enough dishes and silver to serve everyone without asking people to bring their own. And the clean-up was a snap with an electric dishwasher on the job.

But the underlying spirit from the year before was still there. The young people were delighted to be in our home and grateful to us for inviting them. My recollections of these happy and deeply satisfying events are filled with remembered warmth and gratitude. They are for me, as they would be for anyone else, the very stuff of pleasant family history.

But there is one element of these celebrations which is uniquely precious to me. My blindness, which to me has become nothing more than one more of my characteristics, went virtually unregarded by the students. I don't mean that they pretended that it wasn't there. They made an effort to move out of my path when I came through carrying food or drink.

But the fact of my blindness was as unimportant to them as it had become to my husband and children. I remember times like these and renew my hope that the time will come when all blind people will know the freedom for which I am so deeply grateful. This, incidentally, is why I believe so strongly and participate so actively in the work of the National Federation of the Blind.

Meeting The Challenge

by Mary Willows

I sometimes ask people (both blind and sighted) to list the problems they think blind people face. One that I think is most critical rarely shows up near the top of the list, but Mary Willows, a leader in the National Federation of the Blind of California, zeroes in on it as she talks about meeting the challenge. Here is what she has to say about how she came to believe in herself:

As a child growing up in Chicago, I suppose I did all the things city kids do: Girl Scouts, baton majorette, cheerleader, something of a cellist, violinist, and otherwise an average student academically. I am the second oldest of six and the oldest of the girls. Fortunately for me, my mother always needed help with housework. So I learned early to be pretty independent. This really paid off for me in high school.

It was during my freshman year that I unexpectedly and suddenly became blind in a car accident. I had thought of one day becoming a teacher, but after the accident,

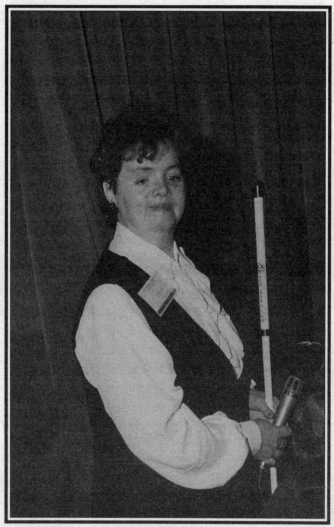

Mary Willows

that just didn't seem possible. I wasn't sure what the future held in store for me. I knew that I had to find something to do with the rest of my life. But what?

As time went on I decided that being a psychologist seemed reasonable and appropriate for me. I liked working with these people and usually developed a good rapport with those I met. Besides, that way I could open my own business and not have to face the rejection of trying to convince an employer to hire me. I just did not believe anyone would want to hire a blind person.

I managed to get a couple of little jobs while I was in college. I stuffed Christmas stockings one year in what I now know was actually a sheltered workshop. I also got a job as a clerk/typist in a company that went bankrupt. So much for that idea. However, I had heard about that job from a blind girl who told me that she knew blind people who were doing all kinds of jobs. "Anything you can think of, there's a blind person probably already doing it," she told me.

She asked me what I wanted to be. Never mind the blindness. I said that I had thought about teaching. She said she knew several blind teachers, and she would introduce them to me. She offered to let me share a room with her at the convention of the National Federation of the Blind in downtown Chicago during July of 1972.

So I went to see for myself. I met teachers, all right. And lawyers, and secretaries and students. Yes, blind students who were pulling straight A's. I met someone who showed me how to use a slate and stylus. He said it was like a pen and paper. It looked like a little metal piece of framework with a hinge on the left. He showed me how to slip a piece of paper inside, close it, and write anything I wanted to in Braille using the notches that were already cut for me in the framework. He used it in all of his classes to take notes.

They used long white canes. They talked about their jobs and their families and their goals for themselves. I was beginning to recognize the challenge, and I started to believe that maybe these things were possible for me too.

I did get my bachelor's degree in psychology, but by that time I was ready for yet another challenge–my master's degree. I still never told anyone that what I really wanted to do was to teach children in a regular classroom, because I didn't believe I could do it. About that time I met Jim Willows, a leader in the National Federation of the Blind of California. We were married and now have two boys.

Children ceased being little creatures from outer space to me. Far from it. I have cared for as many as seven at a time in my home. I learned to believe in myself by putting one foot in front of the other. That little flicker had become a burning flame. I was ready to accept the challenge of returning to school for my elementary teaching credential.

I identified three areas of concern for myself: how to get around independently in an unfamiliar environment; how to write things down quickly for later use; and how on earth was I going to control thirty-three youngsters. I believe in taking one step at a time and solving problems as they occur.

My first action as soon as I knew the name of the school where I would be doing student teaching was to investigate the grounds. I recalled that I knew a blind child who attended that school so I asked her to be my mobility instructor for the day. She was pleased and proud to give me the grand tour.

Many schools in California are made up of small buildings called pods. Since I did not know the classroom I would be in, we located all the rooms. We even found the janitor's office. She showed me where assemblies were held, where the library was located, and how to find the swings on the playground. Since I did not know which grade level I would be working with, it was impossible to obtain any of the texts in advance.

When the time came for me to begin teaching lessons, I prepared myself with Braille notes. I used a slate and stylus for any last-minute instructions from the teacher who was supervising my work. I scheduled ample readers in the evenings so I could preview material for the next day.

If there were papers to collect after a lesson, I put them into a file folder with my Braille notes so that I knew what those papers were. That evening I directed a reader in correcting the papers.

Long white cane in hand, slate and stylus in my backpack, I set out finally to become an elementary school teacher. On my first day of student teaching, my heart was pounding. There I was standing in front of a class of thirty-three very intimidating fourth graders.

My master teacher suggested that I take the children one at a time to the back of the room and let them interview me. They could ask me anything they wanted to know. So I did, and they did. They wanted to know about my slate and stylus. So I decided to seize the opportunity and slipped two 3 by 5 cards inside and wrote each child's name while we were talking.

By the end of forty minutes I not only had all their names written in Braille, but I also had time to connect names with voices. Within my first week, I became responsible for the weekly spelling tests.

I also supervised reading and math groups. Each week the teacher read the spelling words to me so I could put them in Braille. This was another time that I was glad I knew how to use a slate and stylus. This is a skill every blind teacher should have.

My third area of concern was discipline. The first time I was left alone with the students, they were all over the place. I could have died because my supervisor was sitting right there. Of course, the other student teachers at the university were having the same problems. The students were having a field day with their new teacher.

Once I demonstrated to them that I could write the names of the guilty on the board, they decided that I was the boss; and they settled down. I do not let my own children get away with anything, so why should these?

The very next day, I was put to the test. I had to take many different reading groups over to the cafeteria to practice the plays they had been learning. I had never been in a play, so this was going to be interesting. I knew I could direct these plays, and I did. I set each group down at the end of the stage and showed them my slate with paper in it. I said I wanted to hear only the actors. If I heard anything else, the guilty person's name would be written down and later copied on the blackboard. There were only two who tested me.

Student teachers typically start off with the responsibility of escorting the class from the playground into the classroom after the morning bell and after recess. This meant locating my students among the nine hundred others. This was no problem, for when they saw me, they all called my name, which made it easy to locate the line. The line of students did not move until I gave the word. I did not give the word until there was silence. Their own teacher was impressed.

Each morning I chose a monitor to assist with the absentee list and the lunch count. I told the monitor what to write on the absentee slip. I had the students look left, and then right, and tell me who was missing. For the lunch count I had them raise hands; the monitor wrote that count.

I hope that sharing some of my techniques might encourage others who think teaching is impossible because of blindness. In the National Federation of the Blind, we say that given proper training and reasonable opportunity, a blind person can compete with sighted peers and do just as well or just as poorly. The real difference is in whether or not we believe in ourselves. Belief in ourselves is the true key to success no matter what the challenge, no matter what the task.

Daddy Read Me

by Bonnie Peterson

If you could change just one thing about your childhood, what would it be? An interesting question and one which you would normally expect to bring a wide variety of answers. But if you ask this question of a group of blind people, you tend to get one overwhelming response: "I wish I had been taught to read Braille." In "Daddy Read Me" Bonnie Peterson expresses the pain and anguish of a mother who cannot read to her three-year-old. Here is what she says:

I teach communications and public speaking in the university system of Wisconsin. I am also blind. Taking notes is, of course, something that is extremely valuable to me. I take notes on a myriad of topics, and I take them in Braille. I use Braille to write notes to myself about grades and other important information concerning my students.

I also use Braille in my home life–writing down appointments and grocery lists and keeping track of my two daughters' schedules. (They have basketball practice, volleyball and soccer games, and gymnastic classes–and I

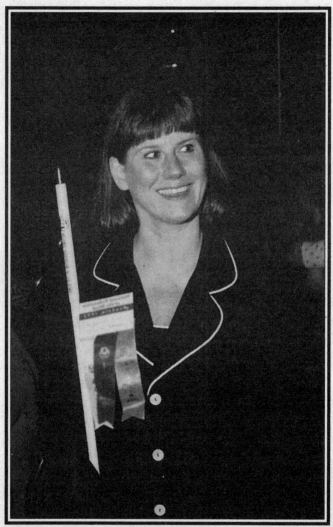

Bonnie Peterson

have to see that everyone gets to the right place at the right time.) But it wasn't always that way. I didn't always take notes in Braille.

When I went to school, my parents were told that I didn't need Braille; after all, I could see. We didn't know about the National Federation of the Blind then. I went all the way through school and college, struggling to try to read with my tiny amount of remaining eyesight.

Then, the National Federation of the Blind came into my life, and I saw wonderful, positive blind people doing things that I couldn't do in a million years–like reading and writing Braille comfortably and easily. These were people who weren't struggling with eyestrain, which had become such an ordinary fact of my everyday life that I didn't even bother complaining about it.

You would have thought that would be enough to make me change, but it wasn't. It took the reaction of my three-year-old daughter to do that.

I was reading her a book about Dumbo the elephant. Of course, reading the book meant wrapping it around my face, straining to see the print, and stumbling as I tried to read what I could not see. I still remember the way she looked at me and said, "Daddy read me." Even though she did not mean to be cruel, what I heard in her words was, "You are stupid!"

That was enough for me. With the help of the Federation, I learned Braille in two months, and my life has been changed forever because of it. Not just because of Braille, but because of the self-confidence I have gained. I owe a great part of who and what I am today to the National Federation of the Blind.

WALKING THE BALANCE BEAM

by Noel J. Nightingale

Noel Nightingale lives in Washington State, where she is a leader in the National Federation of the Blind. A recent law school graduate, she has passed the bar and has secured her first job as an attorney with a large and prestigious law firm. In "Walking The Balance Beam," Noel deals with doubts about her ability to compete in the corporate world—both her own doubts and those of her colleagues. Here is what she has to say:

I am a lawyer with the large West Coast law firm of Heller, Ehrman, White, and McAuliffe. I work in the Seattle office in the Environmental Practice Group. I got the job the ordinary way that new attorneys get jobs with law firms, which is that I worked with Heller, Ehrman during the summer, and they liked my work and offered me a permanent position.

After the bar examination last summer I attended one of the National Federation of the Blind training centers, where I learned

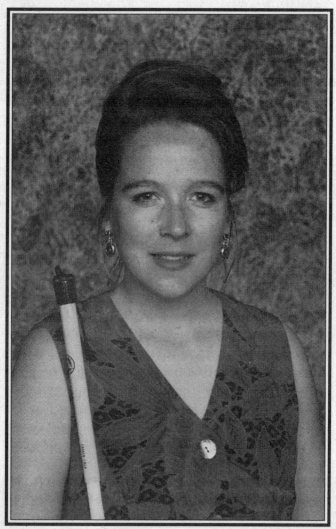

Noel J. Nightingale

Braille and better cane travel and engaged in other activities that helped build my confidence as a blind person.

My job is probably not very interesting to those who observe it from the outside. I research specific legal issues and then write memoranda to more senior attorneys about those issues. I then discuss my research with them and do follow-up research as needed.

As a new attorney I don't get much contact with the clients; I'm pretty much stuck off in my office doing research and writing.

The job accommodations I use aren't unique. I use Braille, a white cane, a reader, and adaptive computer equipment. I find that the most challenging aspect of my job as an attorney has nothing to do with the job accommodations I make. Instead, it's dealing with my colleagues and persuading them to see me as just another new attorney, rather than focusing on my blindness.

Their attitudes and reactions toward me are typified by a retreat I went to with them. It was in a town a little way from where I live.

My law firm had hired an organization which provides business with challenging activities for executives to engage in that are designed to facilitate personal and team growth. We weren't told what these activities would be, and, as the time for the retreat drew nearer, all of the attorneys' anxiety levels about it grew stronger and stronger.

About a week before the retreat one of my colleagues, a friend in the firm who was on the retreat committee, came to me and asked if I was planning on participating in the retreat. I told her that I was, and she asked if I had any concerns.

I said that I didn't know what was going to happen and that I was planning to give everything the old college try. Then I addressed her real question, which was, because I am blind, could I do it?

She assured me that that hadn't been *her* question, but that unnamed people had come to her with concerns about my ability to participate. I said again that I planned to take part in all the events.

But as the retreat drew nearer and nearer, I started hearing rumors about what these events were, and one of them was that there was going to be a very high balance beam that we were going to walk on. I did become a little nervous at hearing that.

The morning of the retreat came and at the breakfast, which all the attorneys attended, the leader came up to me and got down on his knees so that his face was very close to mine as I sat in my chair, and he spoke to me in the kind of voice that one uses in speaking to a child. He asked me if I was really going to participate. I think he was hoping I was going to say no. But I assured him that I was, and he walked away disappointed.

We walked down to the area where we were going to do warm-up exercises, and all went fine until a little way into the exercises. Then they told us to stand on one foot with the other foot touching our behinds. I started wobbling the minute I did it. I had to keep touching the ground with my raised foot. That shook my confidence. I thought, *"If I can't stand on one foot, how am I going to walk on a balance beam?"*

Then I remembered Dr. Jernigan's talking about a sighted person's asking him about a blind person's ability to balance. He tried standing on one foot and found that he couldn't do it very well. But when he practiced a little, he could do it fine, and that steadied me. I told myself that I wasn't balancing well because I was nervous.

We then split up into teams of three and went to the event area. As the sight was described to me, there was indeed a balance beam about seventy feet in the air, stretched between two trees, with a rough ladder against one tree, leading up to the beam.

The leader told us that we would be wearing harnesses with ropes attached to them and that the event would be perfectly safe if we chose to participate. One brave attorney decided to go first. She climbed up and walked out to the middle, where we were supposed to trust those ropes and jump off.

She did just fine, and several more attorneys went, and soon there were only a few of us left who hadn't done it. And some of them were so scared they were talking about not doing it.

I decided that, before these people psyched me out, I had better get going. So I started up the ladder, which was easy. I just found each rung with one hand and then pulled myself up another step. But, when I got to the beam, which took forever, I got myself onto it and put my back to the tree with my hands behind me, hugging the tree. That's when I noticed that the beam was round and narrow-three and a half inches across. I was very scared! So I shouted down to the leader, *"Now what?"*

He shouted back, *"Walk to the middle and jump off."*

I said, *"How?"* Eventually I made myself take that first tentative step, but it was so scary that I quickly jumped back and hugged the tree. I could not figure out how I was going to do this. I stood there for a while slowly realizing that I either had to go or come back down. I was afraid that I would take one step, fall off, and bang into the tree.

But eventually I decided that the best thing was just to get it over with. So I started walking, and eventually I got to the middle. But when they started shouting that I was in the middle, I didn't believe them. I thought they were just saying that to make me feel good. So I kept going. Then I noticed that their shouts were sounding very insistent. It was definitely time to jump.

I stopped and gathered myself for a minute, and then I jumped, and the rope stopped me the way it was supposed to. When I eventually got to the ground, my colleagues rushed up to me and hugged me and cheered. They told me how great I had done, better than anybody else. But I hadn't done better than anybody else. I probably did worse than anybody else, except for the ones who didn't attempt it.

The next two events went fine. I performed at about the same level as my colleagues, or maybe a little worse, or a little better. I don't know. But by the end of the day, I was getting an incredible amount of praise and adulation.

People from other groups were walking up to me and telling me that they had heard that I was the star of the show. I began to feel very uneasy and uncomfortable. Why were these people so impressed by my mediocre achievements? I concluded it was because they had started out with such low expectations of what I was going to do that day. And that very much disturbed me. If they had such profound doubts about my ability to walk on a balance beam, how could they possibly believe that I was able to be as competent at the law as they were?

This brings me to the one other job accommodation I make that I think every blind person must use. It makes all the other accommodations work. I strive to maintain a high level of confidence in myself. The only way my colleagues can learn to have confidence in me is for me to have confidence in myself. But this confidence must be grounded in substance—confidence in my strong blindness skills and in my lawyering skills.

I have heard Marc Maurer, President of the National Federation of the Blind, say that when he faces something challenging, he remembers his brothers and sisters in the Federation and their love and support for him.

That's exactly what I did on the balance beam. After I took that first failed step, I stood up there on that beam and thought about how my friends in the Federation would be cheering for me and supporting me. That's what gave me the courage to go for it and prove that I could do it. That's the only way I know of to maintain a steady level of self-confidence in a world filled with doubts about the ability of blind people.

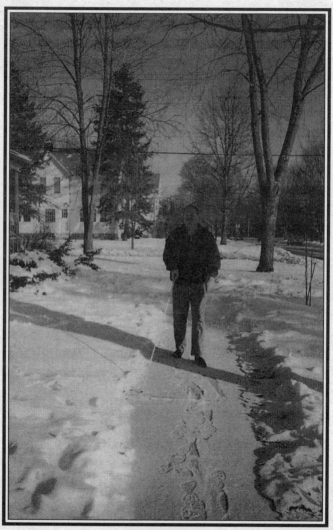

Doug Elliott

Big Enough To Ride The Bike

by Doug Elliott

Doug Elliott lives in Iowa–having moved there from Nevada, where he was president of the National Federation of the Blind of Nevada. In the following story he revisits a familiar Kernel Book theme: What, beyond the traditional "blindness skills" is required truly to overcome the limitations imposed by blindness? Here is how Doug answers that question:

One of my earliest memories is of my fourth birthday when my parents gave me a new shiny red bicycle. The bike was medium sized, but it was still too big for a four-year-old. My father tried to adapt it by making training wheels for the back wheel and made blocks for the pedals so that I could reach them. The training wheels caused me to lean either to the right or left of center, and the pedal blocks would spin instead of remaining steady when I pushed them.

I soon lost interest in trying to learn how to ride my new bike. My father removed all the adaptive equipment and told me I could learn how to ride when I was big enough. When I would see other kids riding their bikes, the image of the shiny red bike would haunt me and soon I was pushing it alongside a rock wall by our house so that I could get on the wall and mount the bike, then push off from the wall. I was determined to be big enough to ride the bike.

At first I would coast just a little and then fall off in the grass. I continued this process, and each time I was going further and further before a crash would occur. Nobody in the neighborhood–parents or other kids–thought this trial and error way of learning was unusual or bad or stupid. Bike riding is a skill that everyone has to learn by making mistakes and falling off. And sometimes you have to grow into it. You have to be big enough to ride the bike. It was frightening to me at first, but I didn't get hurt, and I did learn to ride before I was five.

When I was twenty-one I went to Viet Nam where I lost my sight due to a mine explosion. I thought I would never walk downtown by myself again, be able to get a good paying job, or be able to go out and have fun as I used to do—in short, that I would never be big enough to ride the bike.

I received what is called rehabilitation training—courses in using a white cane and reading Braille, and instruction in typing, cooking, and the use of power tools—skills we need as blind people to live independently. I technically learned these skills in the same way I technically was riding my bike when I coasted a few feet on the grass. But, when I completed my training, I knew that something was missing. I still was just coasting, not really using the skills.

I now know that I was not limited by the fact that I could not see; I was limited by my lack of belief in my own capabilities, my belief that I wasn't big enough to ride the bike. And, of course, I thought other blind people were just as limited as I was. I wouldn't have admitted this; I just knew it inside myself.

When I returned home with my new skills, I found that unlike the experience of learning to ride a bike, the people around me did not believe that the skill of using a white cane should be practiced and perfected. They did not think it would ever be safe for me to walk around freely with a white cane. Neither did I. I was just coasting, not big enough to ride the bike.

My old boss at Sears would not hire me to do the same appliance repair job I had held before going to Viet Nam. He said I couldn't do the job because I couldn't drive to homes where repairs were needed. But he wouldn't hire me to repair appliances in the shop, either.

He knew I could do the work, but he didn't think I could get around the shop safely. He hired me back, but the only job he offered was sitting in a chair all day selling soap and maintenance agreements over the phone. I did this for a little while, but I felt my skills and talents were not being challenged, that I was not really riding the bike.

So I quit.

I knew I was missing something–skills, training, challenges, something. I applied for admission to college and was accepted under probation because they didn't think I could ride the bike. I did the work successfully, earning my bachelor's degree and then master's degree in social work and have worked for the past two decades as a licensed clinical social worker. But, for about half that time, I knew something was missing.

Twenty years after I lost my sight, a member of the National Federation of the Blind invited me to a Federation meeting. I agreed to go but said I was probably not interested because, after all, what could a bunch of blind people offer me? But I went. Afterward, I said to myself, "*This is what I have been missing.*" These people believe in themselves. They are big enough to ride the bike. The Federation message to blind people is that, yes, you will make mistakes and need to practice when learning blindness skills just like everyone practices riding a bike, but that is no reason to stop trying to learn.

When I finally got the Federation message, I started using my cane on a regular basis, started to practice up on my Braille skills, and started to see myself as a capable human being again.

I now know that, before I met the Federation, I was really going through life thinking that sight was the only way to do things. The Federation provided the missing piece–the strong belief that there are other ways than with sight to do things safely and efficiently. If you have sight, that's the easiest way. If you don't, there are other ways.

This simple but vital perspective straightened out lots of puzzles for me and gave me the confidence that merely learning a skill could not. After joining the Federation, I started practicing cane use and Braille reading with a new view–these work for other people, and I can make them work for me.

I recently got married and moved to a small town in Iowa where my wife has lived for some time. My wife has been in the NFB for a long time and has set the norm in this town that the blind aren't helpless and can learn with some assistance.

One cold and snowy winter night shortly after I arrived here, I got lost–completely turned around. Cars passed back and forth but no one stopped to ask if I was okay or to offer assistance as they would have done where I lived before. And I had no idea how to get home. So, I walked out into the street and waved down a car to ask where Broad Street was.

The driver turned out to be the owner of the jewelry store in town where my wife had purchased my wedding ring. He didn't get out of his car or offer a ride home as I expected. Instead, he told me to go one block behind me and turn left–that was Broad Street. I thanked him and left.

The next day my wife stopped at the jewelry store. The owner told her that I had waved him down the night before when I was lost. He said to her that I would have to work on finding my way around here and that he knew he shouldn't give me a ride but rather should give me information, because I would learn faster that way.

With support for each other and the understanding of our sighted friends like the jewelry store owner, we can go beyond coasting, beyond mere skills–to walking outside and going where we want. It's really as easy as that.

I learned it when I was four pushing off of the wall to get my bicycle started. I learned it again on the battlefields of Viet Nam. And I learned it once more when I got home and began dealing with blindness. Maybe all of us have to learn it over and over throughout our lives. The problems may seem to be too hard to solve, but if we work at it with determination and if we believe in ourselves and in the innate goodness of the people around us, we will be big enough to ride the bike.

You can help us spread the word...

... about our Braille Readers Are Leaders contest for blind schoolchildren, a project which encourages blind children to achieve literacy through Braille.

... about our scholarships for deserving blind college students.

... about Job Opportunities for the Blind, a program that matches capable blind people with employers who need their skills.

... about where to turn for accurate information about blindness and the abilities of the blind.

Most importantly, you can help us by sharing what you've learned about blindness in these pages with your family and friends. If you know anyone who needs assistance with the problems of blindness, please write:

Marc Maurer, President
National Federation of the Blind
1800 Johnson Street, Suite 300
Baltimore, Maryland 21230-4998

Other Ways You Can Help the National Federation of the Blind

Write to us for tax-saving information on bequests and planned giving programs.

OR

Include the following language in your will:

"I give, devise, and bequeath unto National Federation of the Blind, 1800 Johnson Street, Suite 300, Baltimore, Maryland 21230, a District of Columbia nonprofit corporation, the sum of \$_____ (or "___percent of my net estate" or "The Following Stocks and bonds:_____") to be used for its worthy purposes on behalf of blind persons."

Your contributions are tax-deductible